Ketogenic Cookbook

Quick Low Calorie Ketogenic Crockpot Recipes with 7 Days Meal Plan

LELA GIBSON

LELA GIBSON

Copyright © 2017 Lela Gibson

CONTENTS

LELA GIBSON

Introduction

I want to thank you and congratulate you for buying the book, *"Ketogenic Cookbook: Quick Low Calorie Ketogenic Crockpot Recipes with 7 Days Meal Plan"*.

This book has actionable information on how to follow the ketogenic diet easily by preparing crockpot recipes.

Many of us want to eat healthy, which perhaps explains the huge number of people who are opting to follow different diets because of the many benefits that they promise. One of the most amazing diets out there is the ketogenic diet, which follows the rule that you should ideally eat more of healthy fats, moderate amount of proteins and very low amount of carbs. This of course means you must take deliberate measures to prepare your own meals to make sure that whatever meals you are eating are low in carb, high in healthy fats and moderate in proteins.

There is a problem to that though; not many of us have a lot of free time to 'babysit' food while it cooks for hours every single day because of our busy schedules. This very aspect can make it very hard to follow the ketogenic diet effectively because think about it; who wants to come home in the middle of the night to start preparing fish and other animal based products for instance, which take forever to cook well when they can just pass by their favorite fast food store or restaurant to buy takeouts?

Well, you don't have to babysit food thanks to the advent of the crockpot. And this book will show you exactly how to make your adoption of the ketogenic diet effortless because all you have to do is put the food in the crockpot then leave it to cook overnight or during the day when you are away to work. And my morning or evening, you can wake up or come home to a hot, home cooked meal! The book has delicious ketogenic crockpot recipes, which you can start making right away.

Thanks again for buying this book. I hope you enjoy it!

Ketogenic Diet For Beginners: An Introduction

What Is It?

As I already mentioned, the ketogenic diet entails eating high amounts of healthy fats and pairing that with moderate protein intake and intake of very low amount of carbohydrates. It is also referred to as the low carb high fat diet (LCHF). Well, although the diet is a low carb diet, this doesn't mean that all low carb diets qualify to be referred to as ketogenic diet. On the contrary, for any diet to qualify to be referred to as a ketogenic diet, it must result to the production of ketone bodies. Ketones are produced when the body starts metabolizing fats into fatty acids and glycerol in the liver after which they (fatty acids) are further broken down into different ketone bodies in a series of metabolic processes. The body opts to burn fat into ketones when glucose levels are significantly low in the bloodstream. So how does this really happen?

Well, I will compare eating the normal American diet which is high in carb with eating a diet low in carb.

When you eat, the different macronutrients are broken down into various forms; carbs into glucose, protein into amino acids and fats into fatty acids. These processes take place in the digestive system before the constituent elements are absorbed into the bloodstream for transportation to different parts of the body. Upon absorption into the bloodstream, the body secretes insulin, a hormone that helps to facilitate the absorption of glucose into the cells for metabolism for use and storage. The purpose of insulin is essentially to act as some sort of 'key' that opens the doors to the cells so that glucose can pass from the bloodstream to the cells. While the process is efficient, there is a problem with this. Given that insulin is secreted in response to rising levels of blood sugar concentrations, if there is an excess blood glucose in the body, a lot of it is converted into fatty acids and glycerol, which are then moved to different fat stores around the body. Well, before the body starts making fatty acids and glycerol, it starts by converting some of the excess into glycogen. But since glycogen stores fill easily (they need just 2000kcal of energy to fill), the body soon moves on to start accumulating fatty acids and glycerol. The more of this you create and accumulate, the more fat you create and the more weight you gain.

The ketogenic diet seeks to reverse that by limiting the supply of glucose (by eating less carb), which in turn greatly reduces the production of insulin. As a result, there is no further glycogen creation and production of fatty acids and glycerol because there is hardly enough to sustain various body processes leave alone store. When dietary glucose reduces, the body starts by secreting glucagon to help in the conversion of glycogen into glucose. The resulting glucose is then used just like any other dietary glucose. But since the stores are limited, the body soon starts looking for alternative sources of energy. With reduced glucose levels coupled with subsequent reduced insulin secretion, the body's ability to burn fat is elevated. This in turn frees up fatty acids and glycerol, which are further broken down into different ketone bodies. Ketones are a great alternative to glucose especially because they are the only replacement to glucose as far as brain fuel is concerned. This is because ketones are water soluble, a feature that enables them to cross the blood brain barrier. As the body burns more fatty acids and glycerol into ketone bodies, this brings about weight loss. As more and more glycogen is used up and the body gets used to using ketone bodies for energy, it gets to a point where it becomes an efficient fat burning machine because it runs mainly on ketones for energy.

For you to achieve that, you have to be deliberate about what you eat to ensure you take sufficiently low amount of carbs to push your body into ketosis. In this case, you ought to eat more of:

- Meats such as chuck steak, bear, pheasant, ham, lamb chops, clams, ground beef, goose, bison, beef jerky, salmon, turkey, elk, ground lamb, lobster, scallops, alligator, veal, rattlesnake, emu, mussel, poultry, venison steaks, beef, kangaroo, turtle, ostrich, goat, quail, sausage, chicken, reindeer, hot dogs, pork and spam.

- Dairy products such as cottage cheese, cheddar cheese, goat cheese, unsweetened plain yogurt, provolone cheese, sour cream, Swiss cheese, ricotta, mozzarella cheese, feta cheese, brie, Parmesan cheese, Gouda, Colby Jack cheese, heavy whipping cream, blue cheese, cream cheese and butter.

- Nuts and seeds such as cashews, pine nuts, walnuts, pecans, hazelnuts, almonds, hemp hearts, almond butter, almond flour, sunflower seeds, macadamia, sesame seeds, peanut butter, pumpkin seeds, Brazil nuts and cashew butter.

- Fats and oils such as animal fats, hemp oil, tea seed oil, flaxseed oil, tallow, pumpkin seed oil, coconut oil, avocado oil, mayonnaise, olive oil, sesame oil, ghee, red palm oil, macadamia oil, butter, walnut oil and cocoa butter.

- Drinks such as herbal tea, club soda, hard alcohol, unsweetened almond milk, seltzer water, dry wines, coffee, water, broth, diet soda, cream and unsweetened tea.

These are great for ketosis since they are low in carbohydrates.

So what can you do to ensure you follow the ketogenic diet effectively? Well, a crockpot can make it significantly easy for you to follow the diet.

Let's briefly discuss some reasons why using a crockpot especially if you are on a ketogenic diet makes your life a lot easier.

✓ *It saves on time*

All you need is the initial prep and your slow cooker will do the rest for you. As your food cooks, you can get lots of things done as you don't have to slave over the pot all through.

✓ *It makes delicious and nutritious meals*

Mostly, fresh ingredients that are cooked for a long period of time under low temperatures are used in slow cooking. Cooking at low temperatures means that the natural, nutrition-and-taste rich juices from veggies and meats are retained.

✓ *Can be used at anytime of the year*

Hot, warm meals are usually associated with wintertime but the beauty of using a crockpot is that it can be used even during hot summers. Slow cookers eliminate the need for an oven during hot times- which makes your kitchen and the whole house even hotter- as it keeps the heat inside the pot.

✓ *Easy and quick clean up*

Aside from the cutting utensils, cutting board and maybe a pan for browning you will only be cleaning just one pot. Amazing, right?

✓ *Saving up on energy*

Crockpots use considerably less energy compared to electric ovens.

✓ *Easily portable*

A Crockpot is easy to move around. You can take it from the kitchen to your office or a party. You just need to plug it in and do your thing.

With that basic understanding, let us now move on to some Crockpot cooking tips.

Crockpot Cooking Tips

When you're using a crock pot to prepare keto recipes, you'd want to get the best out of the experience. The below recipes will help you achieve this

Plan your meals

The crock-pot is a useful tool when you want to leave your food cooking as you go about your day. This usually means turning it on in the morning after you've put in the ingredients. As you can imagine, you may not have enough time to prepare all your ingredients in the morning. Thus, you may need to spend a bit of time in the evening to measure out ingredients and to chop vegetables and meat. This way, you can refrigerate the ingredients separately and place them in your crock-pot in the morning. This will make your work easier.

Meal planning also goes hand in hand with the ketogenic diet. This is because the diet is quite specific when it comes to the foods you need to eat. When you plan your meals, it is highly unlikely that you will eat something you are not supposed to eat because you have everything figured out.

Don't overfill your crock pot

There is one main rule when it comes to placing food inside the Crock-pot. You should not overfill your crock-pot. Instead, only fill it two thirds full. You want your food to Cook properly and retain its flavors. If you give your good some room to breathe, you'll achieve the best results.

It would also help to use the size of crock-pot recommended in recipes. This is because many cooks measure ingredients according to the size of crock-pot they are likely to use. If you use a smaller or larger crock-pot, the results may differ. You may have to do some adjustments in order to get the desired results.

Put just enough liquid

You also need to be careful when it comes to adding liquid in your crock-pot. You should put just enough liquid to cover whatever you are cooking if that's what the recipe calls for. If you put too much liquid, the liquid may start leaking out and this won't be a pretty sight. If you want to cook standard recipes in your crock-pot, try to reduce the amount of liquid by two thirds. This way, your food will cook properly as none of the liquid will leak out.

Layer the food properly

When you layer food in your crock-pot, you should keep in mind that the source of heat is at the bottom. This means you need to place the ingredients that will need more time to cook at the bottom before adding other ingredients. Things such as meat should be placed at the bottom. This way, you can later add vegetables on top if you wish, as vegetables often need to cook for shorter periods as they tend to wilt quickly. Actually, it is usually much better to add the vegetables at the end of cooking, as the heat in the food is enough to cook the vegetables. If not, you will only need to put in the vegetables, stir and cook for a few minutes like 2-3 minutes, and then you remove them from the Crockpot. This will help you avoid overcooking the vegetables.

Don't peek!

It is tempting to keep peeking in your crock-pot to see if the food is cooking properly. This is especially so when you're trying out new recipes. But this is one habit you need to stop. This is because opening the lid often sets cooking time back. This means your food won't be ready when it should be. If you're really anxious about the food, you can check on it during the last few minutes. But be prepared to add a few more minutes to the cooking time if need be. As you become more comfortable with your crock-pot, the need to keep peeking will lessen.

Use your crock-pot to cook various meals

Your crock-pot should not just be used to make dinner. You can also use it to make breakfast, snacks and desserts. You can cook certain recipes overnight and have a tasty meal waiting for you in the morning. You can use your crock-pot to make desserts. You can even use it to brown things such as meat instead of using a saucepan. The important thing is to make use of your crock-pot as often as possible in order to become comfortable using it.

Learn your crock-pot

Crock-pots tend to be different. You may be excited to try out a recipe only to be disappointed when it doesn't come out the way you want. This is often because some crock-pots may take longer to cook the same foods. Therefore, it is advisable to experiment with things such as cooking time and temperature. Check to see if a recipe calls for more time or less time and adjust accordingly. Also, try increasing or decreasing the temperature, to see if the results would be what you want. Once you familiarize yourself with your crock-pot, you will be more confident about trying out various recipes.

Let's now move on to discuss the different recipes you can prepare in your Crockpot while on the ketogenic diet.

Breakfast Recipes

Sausage and Egg Breakfast Casserole

Nutritional info: 484 Calories, 38.86g Fat, 5.39g Carb, 26.13g Protein

Servings: 6 to 8

Ingredients

2 cloves garlic- minced

¼ teaspoon pepper

10 eggs

1 cup shredded Cheddar- divided

1 12-ounce package Jones Dairy Farm Little Links- cooked and sliced

¾ cup whipping cream

½ teaspoon salt

1 medium head broccoli- chopped

Instructions

Take a 6 quart slow cooker and grease its ceramic interior well.

Layer half of the sausage, half of the cheese and half of the broccoli inside the slow cooker and repeat this with the rest of the halves of the broccoli, cheese and sausage.

Whisk together the eggs, garlic, pepper, whipping cream and salt in a large bowl until well combined. Pour it over the ingredients in the slow cooker.

Cover then cook on the low setting for 4 to 5 hours or on high for 2 to 3 hours until set in the center and browned on the edges.

Mexican Breakfast Casserole

Nutrition Information: 320 Calories, 24.1g Fat, 5.2g Carb, 17.9g Protein

Servings: 10

Ingredients

10 eggs

¼ teaspoon pepper

½ teaspoon coriander

1 cup Pepper Jack cheese or cheese of choice

1 teaspoon cumin

1 teaspoon chili powder

1 cup salsa

¼ teaspoon salt

½ teaspoon garlic powder

12 ounces Jones Dairy Farm Pork Sausage Roll

1 cup milk (ideally 1%)

Optional toppings: Avocado, sour cream, cilantro, salsa

Instructions

Cook the pork sausage in a large skillet over medium heat until no longer pink. Add in the salsa and seasonings and let cool.

In a different bowl, mix the milk and eggs. Add in the cooked pork into the eggs then add the cheese and stir to mix well.

Grease the bottom of your crockpot and add in the mixture. Cover and cook on low for 5 hours or on high for 2 ½ hours.

Serve right away with the optional toppings if desired.

Pumpkin Pecan Spice Cake

Nutritional info: 344 Calories, 30.38g Fat, 4.42g Carb, 8.26g Protein

Servings: 10

Ingredients

2 teaspoon baking powder

1 teaspoon vanilla extract

¼ cup unflavored whey protein powder

¼ cup butter- melted

1/3 cup coconut flour

1 ½ cups raw pecans

1 ½ teaspoon ground cinnamon

1 teaspoon ground ginger

¼ teaspoon salt

¾ cup Swerve Sweetener

¼ teaspoon ground cloves

4 large eggs

1 cup pumpkin puree

Instructions

Line a 6 quart slow cooker with parchment paper or grease the ceramic liner using oil.

In a high powered blender or food processor, grind the pecans to a coarse meal but don't turn them into batter.

Add the pecans to a bowl and add in the coconut flour, sweetener, baking powder, salt, cloves, cinnamon, ginger and whey protein and whisk to combine.

Add in the vanilla, butter, pumpkin puree and butter and stir until well combined.

Spread this mixture into the slow cooker and set it on low. Cook for about 2 ½ to 3 hours or just until set and top is barely firm to touch. Serve with coffee.

Breakfast Casserole

Nutritional info: 443.6 Calories, 6.05g Carbs, 18.1g Protein, 38.25g Fat

Servings: 8

Ingredients

1 diced green bell pepper

1 medium diced sweet yellow onion

1-1/2 cups sliced fresh mushroom

1-1/2 cups fresh spinach

2 cups shredded Monterrey Jack cheese

1/2 cup chopped Feta cheese (or other sharp cheese)

12 ounce package of bacon slices, crumbled, cooked and drained

1 cup heavy white cream

1 dozen eggs

1-1/2 teaspoons pepper

1 pound of ground sausage, cooked and drained

1 teaspoon salt

4 cups daikon radish hashed browns or hashed brown jicama (optional)

Instructions

Take a 4 to 6 quart slow cooker and place a layer of the hashed browns at the bottom. Follow with a layer of sausage and bacon and then green pepper, onions, mushrooms, spinach and cheese.

In a different bowl, beat together the cream, pepper, eggs and salt.

Pour this mixture over the contents of the crock pot and cover. Cook on low for 10 to 12 hours. Keep warm in crockpot or refrigerate until when ready to serve!

Clam Chowder

Nutrition Information: 427Calories, 33g Fat, 5g Carb, 27g Protein:

Servings: 8 cups

Ingredients

1 teaspoon ground thyme

2 - 3 cans of fancy whole baby clams (with juice)

1 teaspoon salt

1 teaspoon pepper

13 of slices bacon, thick cut

1 cup chopped onion

2 cups chicken broth

2 cups heavy whipping cream

1 cup chopped celery

Instructions

Cook the bacon until crispy (keep the bacon grease in the pan).

Chop the celery and onions and add them to the bacon grease. Cook until soft (still, don't discard the bacon grease as it will cook with the veggies in the crockpot).

Once the veggies are soft, add all the ingredients (together with the cooked bacon) into the crockpot.

Cook on high for 2 hours or on low for 4 to 6 hours. Serve when done!

Main Dishes

Buffalo Chicken Soup

Nutritional info: 523 Calories, 44.2g Fats, 3.4g Carbs, 20.8g Protein

Servings: 5

Ingredients

¼ Teaspoon Xanthan gum

3 chicken thighs- deboned and sliced (1.2 pounds without bones)

Salt and pepper to taste

1 teaspoon onion powder

½ teaspoon celery seed

¼ cup butter

1/3 - ½ cup frank's hot sauce (as desired)

1 cup heavy cream

3 cups beef broth

2 ounces cream cheese

1 teaspoon garlic powder

Instructions

Debone your chicken and chop it up into chunks and add them to the crockpot. Toss in the rest of the ingredients except the Xanthan gum, cream and cheese.

Set the crockpot on high for 3 hours or on low for 6 hours and allow to cook completely before removing.

When done, take the chicken out of the crockpot and use a fork to shred it up.

Add in the gum, cream and cheese to the crockpot and use an immersion blender to mix up the liquids together.

Add the chicken back to the crock pot and stir well.

Taste your soup and adjust the hot sauce, salt and pepper as desired. Enjoy!

Crock Pot Pizza

Nutritional Information: 487 Calories, 5.6g Carb, 37g Fat, 30g Protein

Servings: 8

Ingredients

3 cups fresh spinach

16 slices pepperoni

.75 pound ground beef, cooked

1-15 ounce jar pizza sauce

0.75 pound bulk Italian sausage, cooked

3 cups mozzarella cheese, shredded

Toppings (optional- you can add your favorites)

1 cup olives, sliced

1 cup mushrooms, sliced

½ green pepper, chopped

½ cup sweet onion, chopped

¼ cup marinated artichoke hearts, chopped*

¼ cup sun-dried tomatoes, chopped*

2 cloves garlic, minced

Instructions

Combine the hamburger and sausage in a 6 quart crock pot together with the onions and sauce.

Add half of the sauce mixture in crock pot and half of the fresh spinach over the sauce.

Add pepperoni and half of each of the desired toppings on top. Place half of the mozzarella on top of the pepperoni and repeat again to end with mozzarella.

Let cook on low for 4 to 6 hours. When done, let cool slightly and slice into 8 parts. Feast and refrigerate the leftovers.

Note

*The marinated artichokes and sun dried tomatoes are not included in the nutritional info.

Chicken Tikka Masala

Nutritional info: 493 Calories, 26g Protein, 41.2g Fat, 5.8g Carb

Servings: 5

Ingredients

Fresh cilantro, chopped (for topping)

3 cloves garlic- minced

2 teaspoon smoked paprika

1 cup heavy cream

1 ½ pounds chicken thighs, bone-in skin-on

4 teaspoon kosher salt

1 teaspoon guar gum

3 tablespoons tomato paste

5 teaspoon garam masala

1 pound chicken thighs, boneless/skinless

10 ounces can diced tomatoes

2 teaspoon onion powder

2 tablespoons olive oil

1 inch ginger root- grated

1 cup coconut milk (from the carton)

Instructions

Debone the chicken on the bone in chicken thighs and cut up all chicken to small bitable pieces.

Place the chicken to your slow cooker and grate an inch knob of ginger on top of the chicken.

Toss in all the dry spices into the slow cooker and add tomato paste, diced tomatoes and olive oil and mix well.

Finally toss in half a cup of coconut milk and combine well. Cook either on high for 3 hours or on low for about 6 hours.

When done, add in the rest of the coconut milk, guar gum and heavy cream and combine well with the chicken (this will help the curry thicken better).

Enjoy with a side of your choice!

Keto Pot Roast

Nutritional info: 307Calories, 0.3g Carb, 13.3g Fat, 2 Protein

Servings: 4

Ingredients

½ cup mild pepper rings (banana peppers)

½ onion- sliced

1 pack dry Ranch dressing mix

Salt to taste

½ cup beef broth

½ cup garlic butter (you can also use 1 stick regular butter plus 4 garlic cloves)

1 tablespoon olive oil

Pepper to taste

1 - 3 to 4 pounds boneless beef roast

Instructions

Sear the beef roast in olive oil in a large skillet making sure all sides are seared.

Place the cooked roast into your slow cooker.

Toss in the rest of the ingredients and cook on low for about 8 to 9 hours or on high for 4 to 5 hours.

Use a fork to shred and serve. Enjoy!

Spicy Beef Soup

Nutritional info: 343 Calories, 22.8g Protein, 1.3g Carb, 25.6g Fat

Servings: 12

Ingredients

½ teaspoon celery seeds

3 cloves garlic- minced

1 teaspoon dill seeds

1 teaspoon coriander seeds

1 tablespoon mustard seeds

2 pounds corned beef- diced

1 pound (453 grams) sauerkraut- the stronger or tangier the better

1 medium onion- diced

8 cups beef broth/stock (homemade, bouillon, or your favorite)

2 tablespoons butter

For topping

Thousand Island dressing

Swiss cheese crisps

To be added an hour before eating

8 ounces shredded Swiss cheese

2 cups heavy cream

Instructions

In a medium pan, brown the onion in a tablespoon of butter over medium heat until slightly golden. Add in the garlic and cook for 1 more minute.

Toss the corned beef, seeds, garlic, beef broth, sauerkraut, onions and the rest of the butter (you can put the seeds in a tea ball if you don't want them in your soup. But they soften up really well).

Cover and cook on high for 3 to 5 hours or on low for about 5 hours.

An hour just before you serve, add in the Swiss cheese and heavy whipping cream.

Serve with thousand island and cheese crisps as desired!

Pepper Jack Cauliflower

Nutritional info: 272 Calories, 21.29g Fat, 6.28 Carb, 10.79g Protein

Servings: 6

Ingredients

1 head cauliflower, cut into 1 inch florets

4 ounces cream cheese

¼ cup whipping cream

2 tablespoons butter

1 teaspoon salt

½ teaspoon pepper

4 ounces Pepper Jack- shredded

6 slices bacon, cooked crisp and crumbled

Instructions

Take a 4 to 6 quart slow cooker and grease its inside.

Add in the cream cheese, butter, pepper, cauliflower, whipping cream and salt and cook on low for approximately 3 hours.

Add in the pepper jack and combine well.

Cook for 30- 60 more minutes or until the cauliflower is fork tender.

Toss in the bacon crumbles and serve!

Caveman Chili

Nutrition Information: 492 Calories, 13g Carb, 35g Fat, 31g Protein

Servings: 8

Ingredients

8 thick-cut bacon

300g yellow onion (1 medium onion)

1 can of diced tomatoes- drained

1 pack of McCormick original chili seasoning

6 ounces tomato paste

300g green pepper (3 small peppers)

2 pounds (32 ounces) ground pork

For seasoning: cayenne pepper, onion powder, garlic powder, pepper and salt

Instructions

Dice the peppers and onions and toss them into your crock pot. Brown the pork and season with pepper and salt and drain.

Let the pork cool and place it into the crock pot.

Chop up the bacon into tiny bits, cook then drain. Let cool and add to crock pot.

Drain the tomatoes and also add to crock pot.

Add in the tomato paste and follow with the seasoning packet.

Cook on the low setting for 6 hours.

Serve when ready.

Low Carb Zuppa Toscana Soup

Nutritional information: 246 Calories, 19g Fat, 7g Carbs, 14g Proteins

Servings: 10

Ingredients

½ cup finely diced onion or 1 medium onion, finely diced

½ teaspoon pepper

3 cups chopped kale

1 teaspoon salt

1 large cauliflower head, diced into small florets

1 pound of Italian sausage, mild or hot ground

½ cup heavy cream

¼ teaspoon crushed red pepper flakes

3 garlic cloves, minced

36 ounces vegetable or chicken stock

1 tablespoon oil

Instructions

Add the ground sausage to a skillet and brown it over medium heat.

Once done, use a slotted spoon to remove the sausage and place it into a slow cooker (at least 6-quart). Get rid of the grease.

Add oil into the same skillet and cook the onions until translucent, for about 3 to 4 minutes.

Add in the chicken/vegetable stock, kale, salt, onions, cauliflower florets, crushed red pepper flakes and pepper into the slow cooker.

Mix well to combine.

Cook on the low setting for 8 hours or on high for about 4 hours.

Once done, add in the heavy cream and mix well.

Serve while hot!

Autumn Beef and Vegetable Stew

Nutritional values: 533 Calories, 39.5g Fats, 9.1 Carbs, 31.9g Proteins

Servings 8-10

Ingredients

2 tablespoon ground cumin

4-5 medium sized marrow squash or zucchini (1 kg)

1 large tin of tomatoes, chopped and unsweetened (400 g)

½ cup ghee, lard or tallow (110 g) -you can make your own ghee

1 teaspoon ground ginger

4 cloves garlic

1 tablespoon paprika

1.5 kg beef braising steaks- boneless (10 medium braising steaks, 150 g each)

1 cup (240 ml) of vegetable stock or broth or water - you can make your own bone broth

1 medium white onion (110 g)

1 teaspoon ground coriander seeds

1 ½ teaspoon salt or to taste (pink Himalayan salt would be amazing)

1 teaspoon chili powder

Black pepper to taste, freshly ground

1 teaspoon turmeric powder

2 bay leaves

2 cinnamon sticks

1 large or medium rutabaga (600 g)

Instructions

Have a 6 quart slow cooker or if you don't, you could halve the recipe to fit a smaller slow cooker. Preheat it to high.

Then use a paper towel to pat dry the braising steaks before seasoning the steaks with pepper and salt (on both sides).

Heat a pan greased with ¼ cup of ghee then add 2 to 3 steaks at a time to it.

Seal the pan until browned all around and when done, add all batches of steak to the heated slow cooker.

Now peel and dice the garlic and onion. Add to a pan greased with the rest of the ghee and sauté until lightly brown and fragrant.

Add in the broth, cumin, chilli powder, turmeric, tinned tomatoes, paprika, ginger and ground coriander seeds. Mix well and cook lightly.

Pour all over the meat in the slow cooker. Add in the bay leaves and cinnamon sticks and cover (cook for 3 hours before adding the rutabaga).

As it cooks, peel and dice the rutabaga. When the meat has cooked for the three hours, push the meat to one side using a spatula and add rutabaga on the other side.

Meanwhile, dice the zucchini and let the slow cooker cook for another hour before adding the diced zucchini in the same side as the rutabaga.

Mix lightly to combine the juices.

Take out the cinnamon sticks and bay leaves using tongs (or just wait until the meal is done) and cook for 2 more hours.

The stew is perfectly cooked if the zucchini and rutabaga are fork tender.

Add to plates and garnish using some fresh herbs such as parsley and cilantro. Season with more salt or pepper if required.

Enjoy!

Cauliflower Chowder

Nutrition info: 205.4 Calories, 14.0g Fat, 11.5g Carbs, 10.5g Protein

Servings: 8

Ingredients

2 cloves garlic- minced

½ teaspoon dried thyme

2 leeks (just whites) - thoroughly washed and sliced

1 ½ cups shredded cheddar cheese

2 stalks celery, diced

4 slices bacon- diced

½ cup half and half*

1 bay leaf

4 cups chicken broth

Kosher salt and freshly ground black pepper- to taste

1 onion- diced

2 tablespoons chopped fresh chives

1 head cauliflower- roughly chopped

Instructions

Place a large skillet over medium high heat. When hot, toss in the bacon and cook for 6 to 8 minutes until crispy and brown.

Line a plate with paper towel and add bacon to it. Set aside.

Add the leeks, celery, cauliflower, onion and garlic into a 6 quart slow cooker.

Add in the chicken broth, bay leaf, thyme and 2 cups of water and mix well. Season using pepper and salt (to taste).

Cover and cook until the veggies are tender for about 3 to 4 hours on the low setting.

Take out the bay leaf and use an immersion blender to puree.

Add in the half and half and cheese and stir.

Serve right away garnished with some chives, additional cheese and bacon if desired.

Note

Half and half is simply equal parts of cream and whole milk. For a cup of half and half, you can alternatively use ¼ cup of heavy cream with ¾ cup of whole milk or 1/3 cup of heavy cream with 2/3 cup low fat or skim milk.

Pumpkin and Coconut Soup

Nutrition info: 234Calories, 21.7g Total Fat, 2.3g Proteins, Total Carbs 11.4g

Servings 6

Ingredients

1 teaspoon garlic crushed

400 ml / 1 2/3 cups coconut cream

½ stick / 55g butter

500ml / 2 cups vegetable stock

Salt and pepper to taste

500g / 1 pound pumpkin chunks

1 medium onion diced

1 teaspoon ginger crushed

Instructions

Add all your ingredients to the slow cooker dish and mix.

Cook on low for about 6 to 8 hours or on high for 4 to 6 hours.

Use an immersion blender with the bald attachment or a stick to puree until smooth.

Keep warm until when ready to serve.

Once ready, garnish with some coconut cream. Enjoy!

Notes

The soup should be thick and heavy.

To make it lower carb, add more liquid to dilute the soup, add more low-carb veggies like cauliflower or serve it as a side dish.

Creamy Beef Soup

Nutritional info: 225Calories, 18.5g Fat, 11.5g Proteins, 4g Carbs

Servings: 14

Ingredients

1 cup sauerkraut

2 large cloves garlic – minced

2 cups heavy cream

32 ounces beef stock

2 ribs celery – diced

3 tablespoons butter

1 ½ cup Swiss cheese - shredded

1 medium onion – diced

1 teaspoon caraway seeds

1 pound corned beef – chopped

¾ teaspoon black pepper

1 teaspoon sea salt

Instructions

Preheat your slow cooker on the high setting.

Add onion, garlic, celery and butter to a large sauté pan and place it over low medium heat. Then sauté the ingredients until translucent and soft.

Add to slow cooker.

Add in the beef stock, sea salt, black pepper, corned beef, sauerkraut and caraway seed to the slow cooker and cook on high for about 4 hours and 30 minutes.

Toss in the Swiss cheese and heavy cream and cook for 1 more hour.

Serve when ready!

Sausage Soup

Nutritional Info: 315 Calories, 7g Carbs, 26g Fat, 14g Protein

Servings: 3

Ingredients

6 ounces smoked linguica sausage- sliced

1 teaspoon xanthan gum

½ cup red onion- roughly chopped

8 ounces sliced baby bella mushrooms

4 tablespoons cream cheese

4 tablespoons heavy cream

1 cup chicken stock

2 medium Serrano peppers- sliced

3 cups fresh baby spinach

To Taste

Salt

Red pepper flakes

Pepper

Instructions

Add the chicken stock and mushrooms to your slow cooker. Season with pepper or red pepper flakes (or both) and salt to taste.

Chop up the Serrano chiles, sausage and red onion and add them into the slow cooker.

Add in a cup of fresh baby spinach and cover. Cook on low heat for 2 hours, stirring only once after an hour.

Add some cream cheese, a cup of fresh baby spinach and heavy cream to the slow cooker and cover. Cook for 1 more hour.

Add the rest of remaining spinach and xanthan gum as desired and cover. Cook for another hour.

You're done!

Paleo Beef Bourguignon

Servings: 6

Nutritional info: 678 Calories, 6.9g Carbs, 36.7g Proteins, 45g Fats

Ingredients

Stew:

8 slices bacon, sliced (240g)

Optional: 1 medium (60g) sized carrot, sliced + 0.7 g net carbs per serving

3 tablespoons ghee or lard (45g)

1 medium white onion, diced (110g)

2-3 large (2 pounds) beef braising steaks, chopped

750 ml bottle dry red wine such as Burgundy

1 tablespoons unsweetened tomato puree (paste)

1 bouquet garni (recipe below)

1 teaspoon salt or to taste (pink Himalayan would be amazing)

4 cups white mushrooms, sliced (300g)

3 cloves of crushed garlic

Optional: ½ - 1 cup water, bone broth or chicken stock if too thick

Bouquet Garni:

3 cloves

1 teaspoon peppercorns

1-2 sprigs thyme

3 bay leaves

1-2 sprigs parsley

Instructions

Chop the beef into large chunks and use some salt to season.

Heat a heavy pot greased with some ghee (around 2 tablespoons) or a Dutch oven. Fry the chopped chunks of beef over medium high heat for about 3 minutes until golden brown.

Turn them around and heat the other side for 3 more minutes. You can work in batches to make sure that the pot doesn't crowd.

Take out the chunks from the pot and add them to a bowl.

Lower the heat and add in the crushed garlic, sliced carrots (if using) and diced onions.

Add back the beef chinks to the pot and add in the tomato paste and red wine (ensure the meat is almost covered)

You can add ½ to 1 cup of broth or water if need be.

Bring the mixture to a boil and stir well so you scrape of any caramelized juices from the bottom of the pot.

Add all of the contents to your slow cooker making sure not to leave out any of the caramelized juices.

To make the bouquet garni- you can place all the herbs in a shred of cheese cloth then tie it up using an un-waxed kitchen string.

Place this to your slow cooker and cook for 6 hours on low or 3 to 3 ½ hours on high.

The meal is done once the meat is tender. Take out the garni.

Now prepare the mushrooms and bacon. Use the rest of the ghee to grease a pan and add in the bacon.

Cook until lightly brown for about 5 minutes and add in the mushrooms. Cook until browned and tender for 4 to 5 more minutes.

Once the bacon and mushrooms are done, take off heat and add them to the cooker with the beef. Mix them well until incorporated.

You can serve over regular keto cauli mash or celeriac cauli mash. Enjoy!

Now that you know what you can prepare with the crockpot to make it easy for you to follow the ketogenic diet, let's put all we've learnt into perspective by highlighting a 7 day meal plan that you can follow.

7-Day Keto Crockpot Meal Plan

Another beauty of slow cooking is that you don't have to cook each meal as you can have food cooking for the whole day and feast on it whenever you want to. The following meal plan is an idea of what you can eat whether in form of a freshly made meal or leftovers. Enjoy!

Day 1

Breakfast

Low-Carb Crock Pot Breakfast Casserole

Lunch

Crock Pot Pizza

Dinner

Slow Cooker Keto Chicken Tikka Masala

Day 2

Breakfast

Keto Crock Pot Clam Chowder

Lunch

Slow Cooker Pepper Jack Cauliflower

Dinner

Keto Pot Roast

Day 3

Breakfast

Slow cooker pumpkin pecan spice cake

Lunch

Slow Cooker Cheesy Spinach Artichoke Dip

Dinner

Caveman Chili

Day 4

Breakfast

Crock Pot Mexican Breakfast Casserole

Lunch

Autumn Beef and Vegetable Stew

Dinner

Paleo Beef Bourguignon

Day 5

Breakfast

Low-Carb Crock Pot Breakfast Casserole

Lunch

Slow Cooker Low Carb Zuppa Toscana Soup

Dinner

Slow Cooker Sausage Soup

Day 6

Breakfast

Slow Cooker Sausage And Egg Breakfast Casserole

Lunch

Creamy Rueben soup

Dinner

Low-Carb Pumpkin and Coconut Soup

Day 7

Breakfast

Keto Crock Pot Clam Chowder

Lunch

Slow Cooker Keto Chicken Tikka Masala

Dinner

Crockpot Buffalo Chicken Soup

I need your help...

We have come to the end of the book. Thank you for reading and congratulations for reading until the end.

There are so many keto recipes options when it comes to slow cooking so don't think that the mentioned recipes are the limit. You just have to be creative. Go wild, mix up ingredients and you never know what you will come up with but first, try out the delicious recipes we've discussed above.

One thing to remember though (as you go wild with exploring), always make sure to keep your meals as healthy as you possible. You are what you eat after all!

Finally, if you enjoyed this book, would you be kind enough to leave a review for this book on Amazon?

I want to reach as many people as I can with this book, and more reviews will help me accomplish that!

If you have any questions or problems, please contact us: hello@freedomdestination.com

Thank you and good luck!

Preview Of 'Smart Fat'

Breakfast Recipes

Coconut-Raisin Quinoa

Quinoa is a food that can be sweet or savory. In this dish, plump raisins and coconut make it sweet while lime zest and cilantro add a savory touch. A dressing keeps the quinoa moist and tender.

Ingredients

Servings: 4

For the quinoa:

1 cup quinoa (well rinsed)

¼ cup raisins

¼ cup unsweetened coconut

1 ¾ cups water

1 tablespoon coconut oil

¼ cup cilantro (minced)

Zest of one lime

For the dressing:

2 tablespoons grape seed oil (or canola oil)

2 tablespoons lime juice

¾ teaspoon honey

¼ teaspoon salt

Pinch of pepper

Instructions

Add the coconut oil to a small pot over medium heat. When warmed, at the quinoa and allow it to toast for 3-4 minutes, until it begins to stick to the pot. Then, the added water and salt to the pot and turn up the heat. Bring the quinoa to a boil and then set to a simmer, cooking for about 20 minutes until the quinoa is fluffy and the liquid is absorbed.

Use a fork to fluff the quinoa and then mix in the coconut flakes and lime zest. Partially cover the quinoa and allow it to sit an additional 10 minutes before transferring to a bowl. Set the bowl at room temperature until cooled.

While you are waiting, whisk the ingredients for the dressing together in a small bowl. You may want to warm the honey slightly if you cannot get it to mix well with the other ingredients. Once cooled, stir in the raisins and cilantro. Drizzle with the dressing and toss to combine.

Barley with Sunflower Seeds and Bananas

This filling breakfast option combines sweet and nutty flavors. The sunflower seeds provide plenty of healthy fat. Since you can make it in the microwave, it is a quick breakfast option that does not skimp on flavor. If you want a softer barley, consider soaking it the night before.

Ingredients

Servings: 2

2/3 cup pearl barley (quick cooking)

1 1/3 cups water

¼ cup unsalted sunflower seeds

2 medium bananas (sliced)

2 teaspoons honey

Instructions

Add the barley and water to a bowl and cook in the microwave on high heat for about 6 minutes, or until done. You may need to adjust this time based on your microwave. Stir the barley and allow it to sit for 2 minutes. When you are ready to eat, top with the sunflower seeds, sliced bananas, and honey.

Cheesy Bacon Quiche

This simple quiche is light, fluffy, and high in the right kinds of fat. A prepared piecrust makes this quick and easy to throw together. You also save time if you use a can of real bacon bits instead of waiting for your bacon to cook before preparing the quiche.

Ingredients

Servings: 6

1 9-inch pie crust (deep dish, unthawed)

1 can (3 ounces) real bacon bits

1 cup half-and-half

4 eggs (lightly beaten)

¾ cup Swiss cheese (shredded)

¼ cup Parmesan cheese (grated)

1 medium onion (chopped)

Instructions

Set the oven to 400 degrees so it can preheat. While you are waiting, add both cheeses, the bacon bits, and the chopped onions to a bowl and mix together. Then, transfer this into the piecrust.

Add the eggs and half-and-half to another bowl and mix together to incorporate. Pour this into the piecrust, covering the bacon-cheese mixture.

Place your prepared quiche in the oven for 15 minutes. Then, reduce the temperature to 350 degrees for 35 more minutes, until the eggs have set and the top of the quiche starts to brown.

Banana Walnut Pancakes

These pancakes have all the deliciousness of banana-nut bread in an easier, breakfast friendly form. They are also a great way to use up your softening bananas before they go bad.

Ingredients

Servings: 3

1 large or 2 small bananas (overripe)

¼ cup walnuts (finely chopped)

1 cup all-purpose flour)

1 egg

1 cup almond milk

3 tablespoons granulated sugar

1 ½ tablespoons butter (melted)

1 tablespoon baking powder

½ teaspoon baking soda

½ teaspoon cinnamon

½ teaspoon nutmeg

½ teaspoon vanilla extract

½ teaspoon salt

Instructions

Add the walnuts, flour, sugar, baking soda and powder, cinnamon, nutmeg, and salt to a large bowl and mix together to incorporate. Then, make a well in the center of the dry mixture.

In a separate bowl, mash the banana. Then, whisk in the melted butter, almond milk, and vanilla extract. Once smooth, whisk in the egg. Pour this into the well you made in the flour mixture and stir to combine, being careful not to over mix.

Add olive oil or cooking spray to a skillet over medium-high heat. Use about ¼ cup of batter to make each pancake. Drop the batter in and tilt the skillet slightly, carefully spreading it around. Cook about 3-4 minutes until the edges become firm and bubbles start to form. Then, flip and cook an additional 2-3 minutes on the other side.

Easy Baked Egg And Avocado Breakfast Bowl

This is a simple, but flavorful recipe. You can serve as recommended in this recipe, or tweak it by adding some of your favorite flavors.

Ingredients

Servings: 4

8 eggs

4 avocados

4 flour or corn tortillas (warmed)

2 limes

1 teaspoon salt

½ teaspoon black pepper

Scallions (optional, sliced for serving)

Cilantro (optional, chopped for serving)

Chilies (optional, sliced for serving)

Instructions

Start by preheating the oven to 450 degrees. Use a sharp knife to cut each avocado in half, carefully removing the pit. Take a spoon and remove about 1 ½ tablespoons of flesh from the avocado, so the opening is large enough that the egg fits in. Cut the limes in half and squeeze each over 2 of the avocado halves, coating with flesh. Sprinkle salt on top and place on a baking tray.

Once all the avocado halves are prepared, break one egg into each. Season with salt and pepper to taste. Be sure to keep the yolk intact, even if some of the white spills over. If you want your avocados presented nicely, consider using a sieve to separate some of the egg white before putting it inside the avocado.

Cook in the preheated oven for 10-12 minutes, until the yolk is runny but the whites are set. Garnish with the toppings and serve with the warmed tortillas.

Bell Pepper Rings With Egg And Cheese

This quick to prepare dish is packed with weight loss promoting ingredients such as apples and kiwi . These are low-carb and low in calories too.

Ingredients

Servings: 2

1/2 medium sweet red pepper

1/4 cup raspberries

2 large eggs (whole)

1/2 kiwi fruit

1/4 small apples

1/4 small bananas

1 teaspoon extra virgin olive oil

1/4 cup shredded mozzarella cheese

Instructions

Cut the pepper into two 1-inch rounds and then put them in a skillet with some oil.

Crack an egg into each ring and cook the pepper and egg mixture for 3-5 minutes until the egg cooks through.

Top with cheese and cover, and let the cheese melt for about 1 minute.

Mix the fruits and serve alongside the pepper rings.

Almond Pancakes

To help promote satiety, add in blueberries, which also promote oral health and are rich in vitamin C. The berries also strengthen your digestive system.

Ingredients

Servings: 4

1/4 cup blueberries, fresh

2 oz. vanilla whey protein

1/3 cup curd creamed cottage cheese

1 teaspoon baking powder

2 tablespoons dry soy flour, whole grain

3 large eggs

¼ cup almond meal flour

Instructions

Mix baking powder, soy flour, protein powder and almond flour. Stir in the cottage cheese and beaten egg.

Heat a large non-stick skillet over medium heat and use canola oil or butter to lightly grease.

Drop the batter onto the skillet, 1/4 cup per pancake. After bubbles start to form flip the pancake and then cook the other side. This should be done in around 2 minutes.

You can serve with blueberries or alternatively add them to the batter before you cook.

Check Out My Other Books

Below you'll find some of my other popular books that are popular on Amazon and Kindle as well.

Alternatively, you can visit my author page on Amazon to see other work done by me.

20 Easy And Fast Diet Tips For Losing Weight – An Easy-To-Follow Weight Loss Guide

Belly Diet: The Zero Belly Diet Step-By-Step Guide Which Will Help You To Lose Your Belly And Enjoy Your Flat Belly

Anti-Inflammatory Diet Guide – The Guide To Reduce Inflammation And Live A Healthy Life Without Pain

Clean Eating: Cookbook And Guide To Restore Your Body's Natural Balance And Eat Healthy

Negative Calorie Diet: Cookbook & Guide Which Help You To Burn Body Fat, Lose Weight And Live Healthy

Smart Fat: Cookbook With Fat Meals Which Help You To Lose Weight, Get Healthy And Improve Brain Function